The Concise Scientific Dictionary

BookCap™ Study Guides

www.bookcaps.com

© 2011. All Rights Reserved.

Table of Contents

A 5

B 12

C 14

D 18

E 21

F 25

G 25

H 29

I 34

K 35

L 37

M 39

N 43

O 44

P 48

Q 55

R 55

S 56

T 60

U 64

V 64

X 65

Z..65

A

acarology [ak-uh-rol-uh-jee] -noun- A branch of the science of zoology which deals with ticks and mites

accidence [ak-si-duh'ns] -noun- The essential parts of a subject

aceology [ase-olo-gee] -noun- Therapeutics, as the remedial way of treating diseases

acology [a-col-uh-gee] -noun- The branch of science concerned with remedies

acoustics [uh-koo-stiks] -noun- The area of physics which concerns sound waves

adenology [ad-n-ol-uh-jee] -noun- A branch of medicine which deals with glands, as their development, structure, diseases, and functions

aedoeology [ey-dee-ol-uh-jee] -noun- The area of science concerned with generative organs aerobiology [air-oh-bi-ol-o-gee] -noun- The science of biological materials that are airborne and how they are dispersed

aerodonetics [air-oh-doh-netiks] -noun- The science of flight by soaring or gliding

aerodynamics [air-oh-die-nam-iks] -noun- An area of the science of mechanics; deals with the way air and gases move and the effects the movement may have on a certain medium

aerolithology [air-oh-lith-ol-oh-jee] -noun- The study of aerolites, which are exceptionally stony meteorites

aerology [air-ol-uh-jee] -noun- A branch of the science of meteorology which involves observing the atmosphere by the use of airplanes, balloons, etc.

aeronautics [air-uh-nawt-iks] -noun- The science of flight and objects that fly

aerophilately [air-oh-fil-lat-lee] -noun- The collecting of airmail stamps or cancellations

aerostatics [air-uh-stat-iks] -noun- The area of science dealing with aircraft which is lighter-than-air agonistics [ag-uh-nis-tiks] -noun- The area of science dealing with public contests or athletic events

agriology [ag-ree-ol-uh-jee] -noun- A comparison of cultures which are nonliterate

agrobiology [ag-roh-by-ol-uh-jee] -noun- The science dealing with the life and nutrition of plants

agrology [uh-grol-uh-jee] -noun- The area of the science of soil which deals mainly with the production of crops

agronomics [ag-ruh-nom-iks] -noun- The section of economics dealing with land and its distribution and productivity

agrostology [ag-ruh-stol-uh-jee] -noun- The section of the science of botany which deals with grasses

alethiology [uh-lee-thee-ol-uh-jee] -noun- The area of the science of logic which deals with truth and error

algedonics [al-juh-don-iks] -noun- The study of pain, especially that which results in pleasure algology [al-gol-uh-jee] -noun- The area of the science of botany which deals with algae

anaesthesiology [an-uhs-thee-zee-ol-uh-gee] -noun- The science that deals with administering a substance which will make the subject insensitive during painful procedures

anaglyptics [an-uh-glip-tiks] -noun- The art form of embossing or carving

anagraphy [an-uh-graf-ee] -noun- The art form of putting together catalogs

anatomy [uh-nat-uh-mee] -noun- The branch of science which deals with the way plants and animals are structured

andragogy [an-druh-goh-jee] -noun- The science of teaching adults and the methods and practices that should be used

anemology [an-uh-mol-uh-jee] -noun- The science behind the way winds move

angelology [eyn-juh-lol-uh-jee] -noun- The scientific theory or doctrine concerning angels angiology [an-jee-ol-uh-jee] -noun- The area of the science of anatomy which is concerned with lymphatics and blood vessels

anthropobiology [an-thro-po-bi-ol-uh-jee] -noun- The study of humans as a species and their biological relationships

anthropology [an-thruh-pol-uh-jee] -noun- A branch of science which deals with the development, characteristics, customs and beliefs of mankind physically, socially, and biologically

aphnology [af-nol-uh-jee] -noun- The area of science which explores wealth

apiology [ey-pee-ol-uh-jee] -noun- The area of science pertaining to bees; honeybees, specifically

arachnology [uh-rak-nol-uh-jee] -noun- The study of the arachnid family, such as spiders, scorpions, mites and ticks

archaeology [ahr-kee-ol-uh-jee] -noun- The study of the cultures of prehistoric people by looking at ancient artifacts archelogy [ahr-chel-uh-jee] -noun- A study on first principles, which are laws that are seen as representing the absolutely highest degree of generalization

archology [ahr-chol-uh-jee] -noun- The study of government and its origins

arctophily [arc-to-file-ee] -noun- The collecting, or extreme fondness, of teddy bears

areology [air-ee-ol-uh-jee] -noun- The study of the planet Mars and explorations pertaining to Mars

aretaics [air-uh-tay-iks] -noun- The science of virtue and the theory that there is no correlation between happiness and virtue

aristology [air-is-tol-uh-jee] -noun- The scientific study of dining

arthrology [arth-rol-uh-jee] -noun- The scientific study of joints within the body

astacology [as-tuh-col-uh-jee] -noun- The biological study of crayfish astheniology [as-tee-nee-ol-uh-jee] -noun- The scientific study of diseases which plague the weak and aging

astrogeology [as-troh-jee-ol-uh-jee] -noun- The science planets and other solar bodies and their composition

astrology [uh-strol-uh-jee] -noun- The study which assumes the heavenly bodies effect human lives and the interpretation of these effects

astrometeorology [as-troh-mee-tee-uh-rol-uh-jee] -noun- The study and theory of the effect that astronomical bodies have on the earth's atmosphere

astronomy [uh-stron-uh-mee] -noun- The science which pertains to the universe that exists beyond the atmosphere of Earth

astrophysics [as-troh-fiz-iks] -noun- The area of astronomy which explores celestial bodies and the way matter and radiation interact within the celestial body and interstellar space in general

astroseismology [as-troh-size-mol-uh-jee] -noun- The area of science that interprets the frequency of pulsating stars to study their internal structure atmology [at-mol-uh-jee] -noun- The science concerned with the laws and phenomena of aqueous vapor

audiology [aw-dee-ol-uh-jee] -noun- The scientific study of hearing disorders, including treatment, impairment, and causes

autecology [aw-tuh-col-uh-jee] -noun- In ecology, the study of organisms within and dependent upon their environment

autology [aw-tol-uh-jee] -noun- The study pertaining to oneself

auxology [awks-ol-uh-jee] -noun- The scientific study of growth, especially pertaining to microorganisms

avionics [ey-vee-on-iks] -noun- The technology of electronic devices as they pertain to aviation

axiology [ak-see-ol-uh-jee] -noun- The area of philosophy which deals with value systems, such as ethical or religious

B

bacteriology [bak-teer-ee-ol-uh-jee] -noun- A area of microbiology pertaining to identifying, studying, and cultivating bacteria and the way this applies to medicine or the environment

balneology [bal-nee-ol-uh-jee] -noun- The study of bathing and its therapeutic effects

barodynamics [bar-uh-die-nam-iks] -noun- The mechanical study of structures which are so heavy they may collapse under their own weight

barology [ba-rol-uh-jee] -noun- The science behind gravity and weight

biology [bi-ol-uh-jee] -noun- The science pertaining to living matter in all its forms, especially concerning origin, growth, reproduction, structure, and behavior

biometrics [bi-uh-meh-triks] -noun- The process of confirming a person's unique traits, personal or other, which will help to confirm identification bionomics [bi-uh-nom-iks] -noun- The study pertaining to the behavior of an organism in its natural habitat and also its adaptation

botany [bot-n-ee] -noun- The area of the science of biology which pertains to plant life

bromatology [bro-muh-tol-uh-jee] -noun- The scientific study of ailments

brontology [bron-tol-uh-jee] -noun- A study pertaining to thunder

bryology [bry-ol-uh-jee] -noun- The area of botany which deals with bryophytes, as nonvascular plants such as mosses

C

cacogenics [kak-uh-jen-iks] -noun- Also dysgenics; the study of the factors which cause degeneration in offspring

caliology [cal-ee-ol-uh-jee] -noun- The study pertaining to birds' nests calorifics [cal-uh-rif-iks] -adj- The generation of calories or heat

cambistry [kam-bis-tree] -noun- The science which pertains to weights and measures or foreign exchange

campanology [kam-puh-nol-uh-jee] -noun- The art of making bells or the principles of bell ringing

carcinology [kahr-sin-ol-uh-jee] -noun- The area of zoology pertaining to Crustacea

cardiology [kahr-dee-ol-uh-jee] -noun- The study of the heart as it pertains to disease and ailments

caricology [kahr-ik-ol-uh-jee] -noun- The study of Carex, a genus of plants which are also known as sedges

carpology [kahr-pol-uh-jee] -noun- The branch of botany which deals with fruits and seeds

cartography [kahr-tog-ruh-fee] -noun- The art of constructing maps, including projection, design, compilation, drafting, and reproduction

cartophily [kahr-tuh-file-ee] -noun- The art of collecting trade cards, such as cigarette cards castrametation [kas-truh-meh-tay-shun] -noun- The art of creating a camp, such as the layout

catacoustics [kat-uh-coo-stiks] -noun- The study of echoes in the science of acoustics

catalactics [kat-uh-lak-tiks] -noun- The science behind the process of commercially exchanging

catechectics [kat-uh-chek-tiks] -noun- The practice of teaching by the use of questions and answers

cetology [see-tol-uh-jee] -noun- The biological study of dolphins and whales

chalcography [kal-kog-ruh-fee] -noun- The art of making engravings in copper or brass

chalcotriptics [kal-co-trip-tiks] -noun- The art of making rubbings from vases

chaology [kay-ol-uh-jee] -noun- The scientific study of the chaos theory

characterology [kair-ak-ter-ol-uh-jee] -noun- The study of character development and character differences between individuals chemistry [kem-uh-stree] -noun- The science pertaining to the composition of some elementary forms of matter

chirocosmetics [ki-ro-koz-met-iks] -noun- The art of manicuring and beautifying the hands

chirography [ki-rog-ruh-fee] -noun- The art of penmanship and handwriting

chirology [ki-rol-oh-jee] -noun- The art of sign language or palmistry

chiropody [ki-rop-uh-dee] -noun- The scientific study of podiatry; the study of feet

chorology [koh-rol-oh-jee] -noun- The study of the cause and effect relationship between certain geographical phenomena occurring within a particular area

chrematistics [kri-muh-tis-tiks] -noun- The study of riches and wealth

chronobiology [kron-oh-bi-ol-uh-jee] -noun- The study of the effects of time and rhythm on living creatures chrysology [kry-sol-uh-jee] -noun- The area of economy and politics which deals with the distribution of wealth

ciselure [si-s-lur] -noun- The art of metal chasing

climatology [kli-muh-tol-uh-jee] -noun- The science dealing with climates and phenomena pertaining to climates

clinology [klin-ol-uh-jee] -noun- The study of the decline of an organism after maturity; aging

codicology [kod-uh-kol-uh-jee] -noun- The study and art of manuscripts

coleopterology [kol-ee-op-ter-ol-uh-jee] -noun- The biological study of weevils and beetles

cometology [kom-uh-tol-uh-jee] -noun- The astronomical study of comets

cryptozoology [krip-toh-zoo-ol-uh-jee] -noun- The study of creatures whose existence is yet unproven, such as the Loch Ness Monster

ctetology [tet-ol-uh-jee] -noun- The study of certain characteristics which are inherited cynology [si-nol-uh-jee] -noun- The study of dogs and the science pertaining to them

cytology [si-tol-uh-jee] -noun- The study of cells under the microscope, such as to check for abnormalities

D

dactyliology [dak-til-ee-ol-uh-jee] -noun- The studying of rings

dactylography [dak-til-og-ruh-fee] -noun- The scientific study pertaining to fingerprints

dactylology [dak-til-ol-uh-jee] -noun- The scientific study of sign language

deltiology [del-tee-ol-uh-jee] -noun- The art of collecting picture postcards

demology [dem-ol-uh-jee] -noun- The scientific study of human activities and social structures

demonology [dee-mon-ol-uh-jee] -noun- The scientific study pertaining to demons dendrochronology [den-dra-kron-ol-uh-jee] -noun- The ecological study of tree rings

dendrology [den-dra-luh-jee] -noun- The ecological study of trees

deontology [dee-un-tol-uh-jee] -noun- The scientific theory of morality

dermatoglyphics [der-muh-tuh-glif-iks] -noun- The scientific study of patters on the skin, such as fingerprints

dermatology [der-muh-tol-uh-jee] -noun- The biological study of skin

desmology [dez-mol-uh-jee] -noun- The biological study of ligaments

diabology [dee-uh-bol-uh-jee] -noun- The theological study of the devil

diagraphics [di-uh-graf-iks] -noun- The art of diagram making

dialectology [di-uh-lek-tol-uh-jee] -noun- The scientific study of spoken dialects dioptrics [di-op-triks] -noun- The scientific study pertaining to the refraction of light

diplomatics [dip-lo-mat-iks] -noun- The study of deciphering ancient texts

diplomatology [dip-lo-muh-tol-uh-jee] -noun- The sociological study of diplomats

docimology [dos-uh-mol-uh-jee] -noun- The art of testing or assaying metals

dosiology [doe-si-ol-uh-jee] -noun- The scientific study of doses and dosage

dramaturgy [dra-ma-ter-jee] -noun- The art of staging dramatic productions and events

dysgenics [dis-jen-iks] -noun- The scientific study pertaining to racial degeneration

dysteleology [dis-tel-ee-ol-uh-jee] -noun- The biological study of organs which have no purpose

E

ecclesiology [ek-lee-si-ol-uh-jee] -noun- The theological study of church functions

eccrinology [ek-rin-ol-uh-jee] -noun- The science concerned with excretions

ecology [ee-kol-uh-jee] -noun- The biological study of organisms interacting with their environment, including with other organisms

economics [ek-uh-nom-iks] -noun- The science of goods and services, such as the consumption and distribution and how it all relates to humankind

edaphology [ed-uh-fahl-uh-jee] -noun- The scientific study of different types of soil

Egyptology [ee-jip-tol-uh-jee] -noun- The anthropological study of Ancient Egypt

ekistics [eh-kis-tiks] -noun- The sociological study of human settlement electrochemistry [ee-lek-tro-kem-uh-stree] -noun- The scientific study of the interaction between electricity and chemicals

electrology [ee-lek-trol-uh-jee] -noun- The scientific study of electricity

electrostatics [ee-lek-tro-sta-tis-tiks] -noun- The science behind static electricity

ephebiatrics [eh-fee-bee-at-riks] -noun- The area of medical science which pertains to adolescents

epidemiology [ep-uh-dee-mee-ol-uh-jee] -noun- The scientific study of widespread diseases, such as epidemics

epileptology [ep-uh-lep-tol-uh-jee] -noun- The scientific study of epilepsy

epistemology [ep-uh-stem-ee-ol-uh-jee] -noun- The philosophical study of the origins of knowledge

eremology [er-uh-mol-uh-jee] -noun- The geological study of deserts

ergology [er-gol-uh-jee] -noun- The scientific study of the effects that working has on human beings ergonomics [er-guh-nom-iks] -noun- The study of humans while they are working

escapology [eh-skay-pol-uh-jee] -noun- The art or study of being able to free oneself from some form of constraints, such as handcuffs

eschatology [eh-ska-tol-uh-jee] -noun- The study of a person's final matters, as in death

ethnogeny [eth-nah-jen-ee] -noun- The study of origins of races or ethnic groups

ethnology [eth-nol-uh-jee] -noun- In anthropology, the study of the historical development of cultures

ethnomethodology [eth-noh-meth-uh-dol-uh-jee] -noun- Studying the use of everyday communication

ethnomusicology [eth-noh-myoo-zi-kol-uh-jee] -noun- The study of the music systems in different cultures

ethology [eth-ol-uh-jee] -noun- The study of behavioral patterns of animals in their natural environment ethonomics [eth-uh-nom-iks] -noun- The study of a society's ethical and economic principles

etiology [ee-tee-ol-uh-jee] -noun- The scientific study of what causes diseases

etymology [eh-tem-ol-uh-jee] -noun- The study of words and their origin

euthenics [yoo-then-iks] -noun- The science of improving life by bettering living conditions

exobiology [ek-so-bi-ol-uh-jee] -noun- The study of life outside of the Earth, as on other planets; extraterrestrial life

F

floristry [flor-iz-tree] -noun- The art of flowers, such as cultivation and sales

fluviology [floo-vee-ol-uh-jee] -noun- The study of courses of water, such as rivers

folkloristics [fohk-law-ris-tiks] -noun- The study of the beliefs or customs of a people futurology [fyoo-chuh-rol-uh-jee] -noun- The study of what may come in the future

G

garbology [gar-bol-uh-jee] -noun- The study of the things people throw away, as garbage, and what it says about society as a whole

gastroenterology [gas-troh-en-tuh-rol-uh-jee] -noun- The study of digestive organs, and their structure, function and diseases

gastronomy [gas-tron-uh-mee] -noun- The art of eating good food

gemmology [jem-ol-uh-jee] -noun- The study gemstones and jewels, both real and artificial

genealogy [jee-nee-ol-uh-jee] -noun- The study of a person's ancestors and where they come from

genesiology [jen-ee-zee-ol-uh-jee] -noun- The science of reproduction

genethlialogy [jee-neth-lee-ol-uh-jee] -noun- The astrological art of writing horoscopes geochemistry [jee-oh-kem-iz-tree] -noun- The geological study of the earth's crust

geochronology [jee-oh-kron-ol-uh-jee] -noun- The study of measuring geological time

geogeny [jee-ah-jen-ee} -noun- Science of the formation of the earth's crust

geogony [jee-ah-jen-ee} -noun- The branch of science which deals with the formation of the earth

geography [jee-og-ruh-fee] -noun- The study of the earth in terms of climate, elevations, populations, vegetation, soil, and other characteristics

geology [jee-ol-uh-jee] -noun- The science which explores the physical history of the earth

geomorphogeny [jee-oh-mor-fa-jen-ee] -noun- The geological study of land forms and how they were created

geoponics [jee-uh-pon-iks] -noun- The art of gardening and farming in soil

geotechnics [jee-oh-tek-niks] -noun- The science of making the earth more habitable geratology [jer-uh-tol-uh-jee] -noun- The study of extinction or the decline of life

gerocomy [jer-ah-kuh-mee] -noun- The area of medicine which pertains to the elderly

gerontology [jer-un-tol-uh-jee] -noun- The scientific study of aging and of the elderly

gigantology [ji-gan-tol-uh-jee] -noun- The scientific and biological study of giants

glaciology [glay-shee-ol-uh-jee] -noun- The area of geology pertaining to glaciers and how their movement effects the topography of the earth

glossology [gloss-ol-uh-jee] -noun- The study of the tongue as it pertains to language

glyptography [glip-tog-ruh-fee] -noun- The art of making engravings on gemstones

glyptology [glip-tol-uh-jee] -noun- The study of the engravings which are on gemstones

gnomonics [no-mon-iks] -noun- The art of using sundials to measure time gnosiology [no-zi-ol-uh-jee] -noun- The philosophical study of knowledge

gnotobiology [no-to-bi-ol-uh-jee] -noun- The study living within conditions that are free of germs

graminology [gram-in-ol-uh-jee] -noun- The branch of the science of botany which pertains to grasses

grammatology [gram-uh-tol-uh-jee] -noun- The study of various systems of writing

graphemics [gra-fee-miks] -noun- The study of the various systems of writing as they pertain to speech

graphology [gra-fol-uh-jee] -noun- The study of handwriting and how it pertains to the personality of the writer

gromatics [gro-mat-iks] -noun- Anything having to do with surveys or action of surveying

gynaecology [gi-nay-col-uh-jee] -noun- The scientific study of the physiology of a woman

gyrostatics [ji-roh-stat-iks] -noun- The laws and study pertaining to rotating bodies

H

haemataulics [he-muh-tohl-iks] -noun- The study of the way blood moves through the veins, and the blood vessels

hagiology [hag-ee-ol-uh-jee] -noun- The study of literature which pertains to the lives of saints

halieutics [hal-ee-yu-tiks] -noun- The scientific study of the sport of fishing

hamartiology [hay-mar-tee-ol-uh-jee] -noun- The theological study of sin

harmonics [har-mon-iks] -noun- The study of acoustics as they pertain to music

hedonics [hee-don-iks] -noun- The psychological and ethical study of pleasure

helcology [hel-kol-uh-jee] -noun- The medical study of ulcers

heliology [hee-lee-ol-uh-jee] -noun- The astronomical study of the sun helioseismology [hee-lee-oh-size-mol-uh-jee] -noun- The observation of the sun's oscillations as a means to study it's interior

helminthology [hel-min-thol-uh-jee] -noun- The scientific study of worms

hematology [hee-muh-tol-uh-jee] -noun- The biological study of blood

heortology [hee-awr-tol-uh-jee] -noun- The theological study of the ecclesiastical calendar and the significance of the historical feats and seasons within

hepatology [hep-uh-tol-uh-jee] -noun- The biological study of the liver

heraldry [her-uhl-dree] -noun- The study of armorial bearings, such as a coat of arms

heresiology [her-uh-see-ol-uh-jee] -noun- The study of any theories which strongly go vary from the teachings of established belief systems

herpetology [her-puh-tol-uh-jee] -noun- The study of amphibians and reptiles hierology [hi-er-ol-uh-jee] -noun- The learning of sacred things

hippiatrics [hip-ee-a-triks] -noun- The scientific study of diseases as they pertain to horses

hippology [hip-ol-uh-jee] -noun- The scientific and biological study of horses

histology [his-tol-uh-jee] -noun- The scientific and biological study of the tissues in organisms

histopathology [his-to-path-ol-uh-jee] -noun- The scientific and biological study of the way tissues change when afflicted with disease

historiography [his-to-ree-og-ruh-fee] -noun- The art of writing about history

historiology [his-to-ree-ol-uh-jee] -noun- The act of studying history

homiletics [ho-mil-et-iks] -noun- The theological art of preaching

hoplology [hop-lol-uh-jee] -noun- The historical study of weapons horography [hor-og-ruh-fee] -noun- The construction of clocks or sundials

horology [hor-ol-uh-jee] -noun- The science which explores the way time is measured

horticulture [hor-ti-kuhl-cher] -noun- The art of cultivating an orchard or garden

hydrobiology [hi-dro-bi-ol-uh-jee] -noun- The scientific study of organisms which live in the water

hydrodynamics [hi-dro-die-nam-iks] -noun- The scientific study of the way liquids move

hydrogeology [hi-dro-jee-ol-uh-jee] -noun- The scientific study of water beneath the ground

hydrography [hi-dro-gra-fee] -noun- The scientific investigation of large bodies of water

hydrokinetics [hi-dro-kin-eh-tiks] -noun- The scientific study of the way fluids move

hydrology [hi-drol-uh-jee] -noun- The geological study of water sources hydrometeorology [hi-dro-mee-tee-or-ol-uh-jee] -noun- The scientific study of the moisture in the atmosphere

hydropathy [hi-drop-uh-thee] -noun- The medical study of using water to treat disease

hyetology [hi-tol-uh-jee] -noun- The atmospheric study of rainfall

hygiastics [hi-jee-az-tiks] -noun- The medical study of hygiene as it pertains to health

hygienics [hi-jen-iks] -noun- The branch of science which deals with preservation of health

hygiology [hi-jee-ol-uh-jee] -noun- The scientific study of being cleanly

hygrology [hi-grahl-uh-jee] -noun- The atmospheric study of humidity

hygrometry [hi-grom-i-tree] -noun- The area of physics pertaining to the measure of humidity

hymnography [him-nog-ruh-fee] -noun- The art of writing hymns hymnology [him-nol-uh-jee] -noun- The theological study of hymns

hypnology [hip-nol-uh-jee] -noun- The scientific study of sleep as it pertains to hypnosis

hypsography [hip-sog-ruh-fee] -noun- The science which pertains to the measuring of buildings

I

iamatology [ey-ma-tol-uh-jee] -noun- The scientific and medical study of remedies

immunogenetics [im-yoo-no-jen-iks] -noun- The medical study of immunity and its genetic connections

immunology [im-yoo-nol-uh-jee] -noun- The branch of science pertaining to the immune system and its structure and function

immunopathology [im-yoo-no-path-ol-uh-jee] -noun- The scientific study of the body's possible immunity to disease insectology [in-sek-tol-uh-jee] -noun- The scientific study of insects

irenology [ey-rn-ol-uh-jee] -noun- The branch of science pertaining to the study of peace

iridology [ey-rid-ol-uh-jee] -noun- The branch of eye science pertaining to the study of the iris

K

kalology [kal-ol-uh-jee] -noun- The branch of science pertaining to the study of beauty

karyology [kar-ee-ol-uh-jee] -noun- The branch of biology pertaining to the study of cell nuclei

kidology [kid-ol-uh-jee] -noun- The area of science pertaining to the study of kidding

kinematic [ki-nuh-mat-iks -noun- The area of science pertaining to the study of motion

kinesics [ki-nee-siks] -noun- The study of communicating by the use of gestures kinesiology [ki-nee-see-ol-uh-jee] -noun- The science which deals with the physiological processes of the body and its anatomy as it relates to movement

kinetics [ki-neh-tiks] -noun- The scientific study of the forces which change the motion of masses

koniology [ko-nee-ol-uh-jee] -noun- The atmospheric study pertaining to pollutants and dust

ktenology [ten-ol-uh-jee] -noun- The scientific process of putting a person to death, such as by lethal injection

kymatology [ki-muh-tol-uh-jee] -noun- The geological study of the movement of waves

L

labeorphily [lay-bee-or-fi-lee] -noun- The art of collecting and studying the labels from beer bottles

larithmics [la-rith-miks] -noun- The scientific study of statistics as pertaining to population

laryngology [lar-in-gol-uh-jee] -noun- The biological study of the larynx lepidopterology [lep-uh-dop-ter-ol-uh-jee] -noun- The scientific study pertaining to moths and butterflies

leprology [lep-rol-uh-jee] -noun- The medical study of leprosy

lexicology [lek-si-kol-uh-jee] -noun- The art of studying words and their meaning

lexigraphy [lek-si-gra-fee] -noun- The art of studying the definitions of words

lichenology [lee-shun-ol-uh-jee] -noun- The study of complex organisms known as lichen, which are fungi united with algae

limacology [ly-muh-kol-uh-jee] -noun- The scientific study pertaining to slugs

limnobiology [lim-no-bi-ol-uh-jee] -noun- The ecological study of organisms which reside in freshwater

limnology [lim-nol-uh-jee] -noun- The ecological study of freshwater bodies

linguistics [ling-gwis-tiks] -noun- The scientific study of all aspects of language and dialect lithology [lith-ol-uh-jee] -noun- The geological study of rocks

liturgiology [li-ter-jee-ol-uh-jee] -noun- The theological study of church rituals and practices

loimology [loy-mol-uh-jee] -noun- The medical and historical study of epidemics and plagues

loxodromy [lok-sah-druh-mee[-noun- A technique or study of sailing along rhumb lines

M

mastology [mass-tol-uh-jee] -noun- The scientific study pertaining to mammals

mathematics [math-uh-ma-tiks] -noun- The systematic study of measurement and relationship between quantities and sets which is expressed by the use of numbers and symbols

mazology [may-zol-uh-jee] -noun- The scientific study pertaining to mammals mechanics [meh-kan-iks] -noun- A branch of the science of physics which pertains to an analysis of the actions of forces on matter

meconology [me-kan-ol-uh-jee] -noun- The scientific study pertaining to opium

melittology [mel-i-tol-uh-jee] -noun- The scientific study which pertains to bees

mereology [mer-ee-ol-uh-jee] -noun- The scientific study of the logic of part-whole relationships

mesology [mes-ol-uh-jee] -noun- The scientific study of ecology

metallogeny [met-l-ah-jen-ee] -noun- The scientific study pertaining to mineral deposits and how they affect the earth's crust

metallography [met-l-ah-gra-fee] -noun- The scientific studying pertaining to metals and their physical structure

metallurgy [met-uh-ler-jee] -noun- The scientific study pertaining to the treatment and alloying of metals metaphysics [met-uh-fiz-iks] -noun- The philosophical study pertaining to the fundamental nature of beings and the world

metapolitics [met-uh-pol-uh-tiks] -noun- A study pertaining to politics, either in theory or in the abstract

metapsychology [met-uh-si-kol-uh-jee] -noun- The study of nature as it pertains to the mind

meteoritics [mee-tee-uh-rit-iks] -noun- The astronomical study of meteors

meteorology [mee-tee-uh-rol-uh-jee] -noun- The area of science pertaining to the climate of the atmosphere and any phenomena associated with it

metrics [meh-triks] -noun- The science of meter as it pertains to music

metrolo [met-rol-uh-jee] -noun- The scientific study of weights and measures

microanatomy [mi-kro-uh-nat-uh-mee] -noun- The scientific study of microscopic tissues microbiology [mi-kro-bi-ol-uh-jee] -noun- The scientific study of microscopic organisms

microclimatology [mi-kro-cli-ma-tol-uh-jee] -noun- The scientific study of climate differentiation in local zones

micrology [mi-krol-uh-jee] -noun- The branch of science which pertains to microscopic things, or things with subtle differences

micropalaeontology [mi-kro-pay-lee-on-tol-uh-jee] -noun- The scientific study of fossils which are microscopic in size

microphytology [mi-kro-phi-tol-uh-jee] -noun- The scientific study of plant life which is microscopic in size

microscopy [mi-kro-ska-pee] -noun- The scientific study of objects which are very small

mineralogy [min-er-ol-uh-jee] -noun- The geological study of minerals

molinology [mo-lin-ol-uh-jee] -noun- The scientific study of milling, or of mills momilogy [mo-mil-uh-jee] -noun- The scientific study of things which have been mummified

morphology [mor-fol-uh-jee] -noun- The biological study of the structure of organisms, not dependent on their function

muscology [mus-kol-uh-jee] -noun- The scientific study of mosses

museology [myoo-si-ol-uh-jee] -noun- The artistic study of museums

musicology [myoo-zi-kol-uh-jee] -noun- The scholarly and artistic study of all things musical

mycology [mi-kol-uh-jee] -noun- The scientific study of the fungi family

myology [mi-ol-uh-jee] -noun- The biological study of muscles and musculature

myrmecology [meer-muh-kol-uh-jee] -noun- The scientific study of ants

mythology [mi-thol-uh-jee] -noun- The historical and scientific study of myths

N

naology [nay-ol-uh-jee] -noun- The artistic study of the architecture of churches and temples

nasology [nay-zol-uh-jee] -noun- The biological study of the nose

nautics [naw-tiks] -noun- The artistic study of navigation

nomology [no-mol-uh-jee] -noun- The scientific study of law-making, especially laws as they pertain to the mind

noology [no-ol-uh-jee] -noun- The scientific study of intellect and intelligence

nosology [no-zol-uh-jee] -noun- The scientific study of diseases and their causes

nostology [na-stol-uh-jee] -noun- The scientific study of mental senility

notaphily [no-tuh-fi-lee] -noun- The art of collecting checks or bank notes numerology [noo-muh-rol-uh-jee] -noun- The study of how a person's birth date, seen in numbers, can affect their life, it's course, and the events which take place

numismatics [noo-miz-ma-tiks] -noun- The scientific study of coinage

nymphology [nim-fal-uh-jee] -noun- The scientific study of nymph creatures

O

obstetrics [ob-ste-triks] -noun- The medical study of a woman's health as it is associated with childbirth

oceanography [oh-shun-og-ruh-fee] -noun- The geographical study of the ocean

oceanology [oh-shun-ol-uh-jee] -noun- The scientific study of the biological and physical aspects of the ocean

odology [oh-doll-uh-jee] -noun- The scientific study of roadways odontology [oh-don-tol-uh-jee] -noun- The biological and medical study of teeth

oenology [oh-nol-uh-jee] -noun- The science of winemaking and all aspects of wine, except the growing process of the vines

oikology [oi-kol-uh-jee] -noun- A study of the art of housekeeping

olfactology [ol-fak-tol-uh-jee] -noun- The biological study of the sense of smell

ombrology [om-brah-luh-jee] -noun- The scientific study of rain

oncology [on-kol-uh-jee] -noun- The medical and biological study of tumors

oneirology [oh-nuh-rol-uh-jee] -noun- The study of dreaming and the meaning of dreams

onomasiology [oh-nuh-maz-ee-ol-uh-jee] -noun- The branch of the study of linguistics which pertains to nomenclature

onomastics [oh-nuh-maz-tiks] -noun- The study of the origins of names and also of proper names ontology [on-tol-uh-jee] -noun- The philosophical study of the nature of being and of existence

oology [oh-ol-uh-jee] -noun- The study of birds' nests

ophiology [oh-fee-ol-uh-jee] -noun- The study of snakes

ophthalmology [of-thuh-mol-uh-jee] -noun- The medical study of the eye, including its diseases, anatomy, and physiology

optics [op-tiks] -noun- The scientific study of vision and also of the properties of visible and invisible light

optology [op-tol-uh-jee] -noun- The scientific study of sight

optometry [op-tom-i-tree] -noun- The practice of conducting eye examinations with the use of certain instruments to check for abnormalities and vision problems

orchidology [or-ki-dol-uh-jee] -noun- The area of the science of botany pertaining to orchids

ornithology [or-ni-thol-uh-jee] -noun- The scientific study of birds orology [o-rol-uh-jee] -noun- The geological study of mountains

orthoepy [or-tho-pee] -noun- The linguistic study of correct pronunciation

orthography [or-thog-ruh-fee] -noun- The art of writing words in their accepted form with regard to usage and spelling

orthopterology [or-thop-ter-ol-uh-jee] -noun- The scientific study of cockroaches

"mineralogy"[min-er-ol-uh-jee] -noun- The scientific study of minerals

osmics [oz-miks] -noun- The study of smells

osmology [oz-mol-uh-jee]-noun- The scientific study of olfactory processes

osphresiology [oz-free-zee-ol-uh-jee] -noun- The scientific and biological study of the sense of smell

osteology [oz-tee-ol-uh-jee] -noun- The scientific and biological study of bones otology [oh-tol-uh-jee] -noun- The scientific and biological study of the ear

otorhinolaryngology [oh-tor-hi-no-lair-in-gol-uh-jee] -noun- The medical and biological study of the ear, nose, and throat

P

paedology [pi-dol-uh-jee] -noun- The study of children in regards to their development, growth, and character

paedotrophy [pi-dot-ruh-fee] -noun- The art of raising children

paidonosology [pi-don-uh-sol-uh-jee] -noun- The medical study of diseases which afflict children

paleoosteology [pay-lee-oh-oz-tee-ol-uh-jee] -noun- The archeological study of ancient skeletons and bones

palynology [pol-en-ol-uh-jee] -noun- The scientific study pertaining to pollen papyrology [pap-uh-rol-uh-jee] -noun- The scientific study of paper, its uses, and its development

parapsychology [par-uh-si-kol-uh-jee] -noun- The psychological study of all things paranormal

parasitology [par-uh-si-tol-uh-jee] -noun- The science and study of parasites and the effects of parasitism

paroemiology [par-oh-ee-mee-ol-uh-jee] -noun- The linguistic study of proverbs

parthenology [par-thuh-nol-uh-jee] -noun- The study pertaining to virgins and virginity

pataphysics [pat-uh-fiz-iks] -noun- The study of what lies beyond the metaphysical; sort of a parody expressed in nonsensical language

pathology [puh-thol-uh-jee] -noun- The science of diseases, including their origin, development, and effects

patrology [puh-trol-uh-jee] -noun- The theological study of early Christianity

pedagogics [ped-uh-goj-iks] -noun- The art of teaching and the study of educating pedology [ped-ol-uh-jee] -noun- The geological study of soils

pelology [pel-ol-uh-jee] -noun- The geological study of mud

penology [pee-nol-uh-jee] -noun- The study of the penal system such has the management of prisons and rehabilitation of criminals

periodontics [per-ee-uh-don-tiks] -noun- The medical science concerned with periodontal diseases in the mouth

peristerophily [per-iz-tuh-ro-fi-lee] -noun- The art of collecting pigeons

pestology [pest-ol-uh-jee] -noun- The scientific study of pests

petrology [pet-rol-uh-jee] -noun- The geological study of rocks

pharmacognosy [far-muh-cog-nuh-see] -noun- The medical study of drugs which come from plants and animals pharmacology [far-muh-kol-uh-jee] -noun- The scientific study of drugs

pharology [fuh-rol-uh-jee] -noun- The artful study of lighthouses

pharyngology [far-ing-gol-uh-jee] -noun- The study of the pharynx and any connected diseases

phenology [fee-nol-uh-jee] -noun- The study of the effects of climate on organisms

phenomenology [fi-nom-uh-nol-uh-jee] -noun- The study of anything which is excessively impressive or extraordinary

philately [fi-lat-l-ee] -noun- The hobby of collecting postal stamps or memorabilia, possibly as an investment

philematology [fil-uh-ma-tol-uh-jee] -noun- A study of the act of kissing

phillumeny [fil-oo-man-ee] -noun- The art of collecting labels from matchboxes

philology [fil-ol-uh-jee] -noun- The study of historical linguistics, as in ancient texts philosophy [fi-los-uh-fee] -noun- The philosophical investigation of the principles of knowledge and reality

phoniatrics [fo-nee-a-triks] -noun- The study of speech defects and the correction of such defects

phonology [fuh-nol-uh-jee] -noun- The study of the sounds of speech in regards to language

photobiology [fo-to-bi-ol-uh-jee] -noun- The study of the way organisms react to sunlight

phraseology [fray-zee-ol-uh-gee] -noun- The study of the way words and phrases are used in language and conversation

phrenology [fren-ol-uh-jee] -noun- The study of a person's character based on the bumps on their head

phycology [fi-kol-uh-jee] -noun- The scientific study pertaining to seaweed and algae

physics [fiz-iks] -noun- The branch of science which pertains to force, motion, matter, and energy physiology [fiz-ee-ol-uh-jee] -noun- The branch of biology pertaining to the functions of living organisms and their parts

phytology [fi-tol-uh-jee] -noun- Botany; the scientific study of plants

piscatology [piz-ka-tol-uh-jee] -noun- The biological study of fish

pisteology [piz-tee-ol-uh-jee] -noun- The theological study of faith

planetology [plan-uh-tol-uh-jee] -noun- The astronomical study of the planets

plutology [ploo-tol-uh-jee] -noun- The study of wealth within the political economy

pneumatics [noo-mat-iks] -noun- The branch of physics pertaining to air and other gases and their mechanical processes

podiatry [puh-di-uh-tree] -noun- The medical study of the human foot and the prevention and treatment of foot diseases prosody [pros-uh-dee] -noun- The study of poetic verses and meters

protistology [proh-ti-stol-uh-jee] -noun- The study of the taxonomic kingdom of protists

proxemics [prok-see-miks] -noun- The study of one's desire and need for personal space

psalligraphy [suh-lig-ruh-fee] -noun- Cutting paper in the form of pictures, as an art form

psephology [see-fol-uh-jee] -noun- The study of the election process

Q

quinology [kwin-ol-uh-jee] -noun- The study of the alkaloid quinine, which comes from the cinchona bark

R

raciology [ray-see-ol-uh-jee] -noun- The study of races and racial differences radiology [ray-dee-ol-uh-jee] -noun- The medical study of taking x-rays and the application of x-rays in the medical setting

rheumatology [roo-muh-tol-uh-jee] -noun- The study of the disorder rheumatism, which causes pain in the back and extremities

rhinology [ri-nol-uh-jee] -noun- The scientific and anatomical study of the nose

rhochrematics [ro-kra-mat-iks] -noun- The science in management, in terms of inventory as well as the moving of products

runology [roo-nol-uh-jee] -noun- The study of runes, which are the characters and symbols in ancient alphabets

S

sarcology [sar-col-uh-jee] -noun- The study of flesh on the body and the areas of the body which are fleshiest

satanology [say-tan-ol-uh-jee] -noun- The study of satan and satanistic activities scatology [skuh-tol-uh-jee] -noun- The study pertaining to obscenities or excrement, and the preoccupation with these things

schematonics [skee-muh-ton-iks] -noun- Using gestures to express one's thoughts, emotions, and actions

sciagraphy [si-ag-ruh-fee] -noun- The art of studying and projecting shadows as they pertain to nature

siderography [si-duh-rog-ruh-fee] -noun- The art of impressive or engraving images on steel

sigillography [sig-uh-loh-ruh-fee] -noun- The study of seals, as impressions, stamps, or engravings

significs [sig-nif-iks] -noun- The science of significance, or of meaning

silvics [sil-viks] -noun- The scientific study of the lifespan of trees

sindonology [sin-din-ol-uh-jee] -noun- The study of the shroud of Turin, which is a piece of cloth bearing the image of a man who appears to have been injured by means of crucifixion.

Sinology [sin-ol-uh-jee] -noun- he study of the country of China and all aspects involved

sitology [si-tol-uh-jee] -noun- The medical study of nutrition and dietetics

sociobiology [so-see-oh-bi-ol-uh-jee] -noun- The study of which aspects of biology affect social behaviors

sociology [so-see-ol-uh-jee] -noun- The science of the way a society functions, such as its origin, development, and organization

somatology [so-muh-tol-uh-jee] -noun- The scientific study of the properties of matter

sophiology [so-fee-ol-uh-jee] -noun- The scientific study pertaining to ideas

soteriology [suh-teer-ee-ol-uh-jee] -noun- The theological idea of achieving salvation through Jesus Christ

spectrology [spek-trol-uh-jee] -noun- The scientific study of ghostly beings stratigraphy [struh-tig-ruh-fee] -noun- A branch of geology which is dedicated to stratified rocks, such as their nomenclature and classification

stratography [struh-tog-ruh-fee] -noun- The study of armies, such as what makes an army or the art of leading an army

stylometry [sti-lom-uh-tree] -noun- Using statistical analysis to interpret and study literature

suicidology [soo-uh-si-dol-uh-jee] -noun- The study of suicide, such as prevention or causes

symbology [sim-bol-uh-jee] -noun- The study of things which are symbolic, such as things which represent something else

symptomatology [simp-tuh-mol-uh-jee] -noun- The medical study of the classifications and symptoms of disease

synecology [sin-i-kol-uh-jee] -noun- The branch of ecology which pertains to the way communities of organisms interact with their environment

synectics [sin-ek-tiks] -noun- The study of invention and the processes which lead to it syntax [sin-taks] -noun- The study of the orderly arrangement of words in grammatical sentences; sentence structure

syphilology [sif-il-uh-jee] -noun- The study of syphilis, as a sexually transmitted disease

systematology [sis-tuh-muh-tol-uh-jee] -noun- The scientific study of the formation of systems

T

taxidermy [tak-si-der-mee] -noun- The art of stuffing and mounting the skins of animals which have been preserved and thereby keeping the deceased animal in a lifelike form

tectonics [tek-ton-iks] -noun- The scientific study of the structural features of the earth, or the construction of buildings

tegestology [te-jes-tol-uh-jee] -noun- The collecting and subsequent study of beer mats

teleology [tel-ee-ol-uh-jee] -noun- The study of a purposeful design in terms of explaining phenomena telmatology [tel-muh-tol-uh-jee] -noun- The geological study of swamplands

teratology [ter-uh-tol-uh-jee] -noun- The study of abnormalities or monstrosities in the formation of organisms

teuthology [too-thol-uh-jee] -noun- The scientific study of cephalopods, such as squid, cuttlefish, or octopus

textology [teks-tol-uh-jee] -noun- The study of how texts are produced

thalassography [thal-uh-sog-ruh-fee] -noun- The scientific study of the sea

thanatology [than-uh-tol-uh-jee] -noun- The scientific study of death and any customs associated with death

thaumatology [thaw-muh-tol-uh-jee] -noun- The scientific study of miraculous occurrences

theology [thee-ol-uh-jee] -noun- The study of religious truths and how the universe can be attributed to God's work theriatrics [theer-ee-a-triks] -noun- The practice and application of veterinary medicine

theriogenology [theer-ee-oh-juh-nol-uh-jee] -noun- The veterinary science concerned with the reproduction of animals

thermology [ther-mol-uh-jee] -noun- The scientific study pertaining to heat

therology [the-rol-uh-jee] -noun- The scientific study pertaining to wild animals

thremmatology [threm-uh-tol-uh-jee] -noun- The scientific practice of breeding animals under domestic circumstances

threpsology [threp-sol-uh-jee] -noun- The scientific study of nutrition

tidology [ti-dol-uh-jee] -noun- The geological study of the tides

timbrology [tim-brol-uh-jee] -noun- The artistic and historical study of postage stamps

tocology [toh-kol-uh-jee] -noun- The medicinal art of midwifery tonetics [toh-net-iks] -noun- The linguistic study pertaining to pronunciation

topology [tuh-pol-uh-jee] -noun- The study of any given place, such as the history of a region and its topography

toponymics [top-uh-nim-iks] -noun- The study of names as derived from certain places or regions

toreutics [toh-roo-tiks] -noun- The study of chasing and embossing artwork in metal

toxicology [tok-si-kol-uh-jee] -noun- The scientific study of poisons, such as detection, effects, and treatment

toxophily [tok-suh-fi-lee] -noun- The art of being devoted to archery

traumatology [trou-muh-tol-uh-jee] -noun- The branch of surgery which pertains to major wounds which are caused by some sort of violence or accident

tribology [tri-bol-uh-jee] -noun- The scientific study of interacting surfaces in motion, such as lubrication, wear, and friction turnery [ter-ner-ee] -noun- The art of using a lathe, which is a device for shaping pieces of wood or metal

typhlology [tif-lol-uh-jee] -noun- The scientific study of blindness and its causes and treatment

typography [ti-pog-ruh-fee] -noun- The art of typing or of printing

typology [tip-ol-uh-jee] -noun- The study of things which have characteristics in common; types

U

ufology [yoo-fol-uh-jee] -noun- The scientific study of unidentified flying objects

uranography [yer-in-og-ruh-fee] -noun- The branch of astronomy pertaining to the mapping of stars and other celestial bodies

uranology [yer-in-ol-uh-jee] -noun- The study of astronomy and of the heavens

urbanology [er-bin-ol-uh-jee] -noun- The study of cities and other urban areas urenology [yer-in-ol-uh-jee] -noun- The scientific study pertaining to rust molds

urology [yer-ol-uh-jee] -noun- The biological study of the urinary tract and of urine

V

virology [vi-rol-uh-jee] -noun- The medical and biological study of viruses

vitrics [vi-triks] -noun- The art of making products out of glass and also the technology involved in such a process

volcanolog y[vol-kuh-nol-uh-jee] -noun- The scientific study of volcanoes

vulcanology [vul-kan-ol-uh-jee] -noun- The scientific study of volcanoes

X

xylography [zi-log-ruh-fee] -noun- The art of making engravings on wood, or of printing from such engravings xylology [zi-lol-uh-jee] -noun- The scientific study pertaining to wood

Z

zenography [zee-nog-ruh-fee] -noun- The astronomical study of the planet Jupiter

zoiatrics [zoy-a-triks] -noun- The medical study pertaining to veterinary surgery

zoophysics [zoo-fiz-iks] -noun- The physical study of animal bodies

zoosemiotics [zoo-sem-ee-a-tiks] -noun- The study pertaining to how animals communicate

zootaxy [zoo-tak-si] -noun- The scientific classification of animals and how this process unfolds

zootechnics [zoo-tek-niks] -noun- The scientific process of breeding animals

zygology [zi-gol-uh-jee] -noun- The scientific study and practice of joining and fastening zymurgy [zim-er-jee] -noun- The branch of chemistry pertaining to the process of brewing and distilling

www.ingramcontent.com/pod-product-compliance
Lightning Source LLC
Chambersburg PA
CBHW071626170526
45166CB00003B/1210